Nuno Menezes Gonçalves

Determining factors in the outcome of surgical recovery procedures

Nuno Menezes Gonçalves

Determining factors in the outcome of surgical recovery procedures

Periodontal Plastic Surgery

ScienciaScripts

Imprint

Any brand names and product names mentioned in this book are subject to trademark, brand or patent protection and are trademarks or registered trademarks of their respective holders. The use of brand names, product names, common names, trade names, product descriptions etc. even without a particular marking in this work is in no way to be construed to mean that such names may be regarded as unrestricted in respect of trademark and brand protection legislation and could thus be used by anyone.

Cover image: www.ingimage.com

This book is a translation from the original published under ISBN 978-613-9-63250-3.

Publisher:
Sciencia Scripts
is a trademark of
Dodo Books Indian Ocean Ltd. and OmniScriptum S.R.L publishing group

120 High Road, East Finchley, London, N2 9ED, United Kingdom
Str. Armeneasca 28/1, office 1, Chisinau MD-2012, Republic of Moldova, Europe
Printed at: see last page
ISBN: 978-620-7-65494-9

To my parents,

Maria da Conceição Menezes and Nuno Gonçalves

To my grandfather,

Fernando Gonçalves

To my grandmother,

Maria do Rosário Aguiar

ACKNOWLEDGEMENTS

In order to write this dissertation, I received the collaboration, dedication and encouragement of several people whom I can only thank:

To Professor Miguel Pinto, my scientific supervisor and professor of Periodontology, whom I would like to thank first and foremost for the interest he aroused in the subject, for the desire he instilled in me to explore Periodontology and for all the trust, inspiration, encouragement and contribution he made in passing on his knowledge to the preparation of this monograph.

To my parents, for all the commitment, support and trust they have placed in me throughout my academic career, and specifically in this project, and for the investment they have made in me. In particular, to my mum, for constantly encouraging me to persevere in the fight for my dreams and to give myself body and soul to my degree.

To my family, especially my grandparents, aunt and uncle and sister, who have always supported me through hard times, celebrated my successes with me and tirelessly encouraged me throughout my academic career.

To Joana, for her understanding, acceptance, help and support, always unconditional, and for accompanying and supporting me in all the good and not-so-good times.

CONTENTS

CHAPTER 1   5

CHAPTER 2   8

CHAPTER 3   10

CHAPTER 4   35

CHAPTER 5   36

SUMMARY

Gingival recession is the apical migration of the gingival margin from its original position at or within a millimetre of the cemento-enamel junction, which exposes the root surface to the oral environment. Its etiology is multifactorial, and the most frequent complaints of patients suffering from this condition are dental hypersensitivity and poor aesthetics. Periodontal treatment of gingival recession encompasses surgical and non-surgical means, with the most effective therapy being provided by the field of periodontal plastic surgery, namely root coverage surgery. Despite the wide variety and adaptability of surgical techniques, the prognosis and success of root coverage surgery depend on various intrinsic and extrinsic factors. In this bibliographical review, we set out to survey the parameters that the scientific literature says have an impact on the course of root coverage, look for their scientific basis and carry out a critical analysis of them.

CHAPTER 1

INTRODUCTION

Gingival recession is defined as the apical migration of the gingival margin from its original position at the cemento-enamel junction or within one millimetre of it, with exposure of the root surface to the oral environment. From a clinical point of view, it is measured as the distance from the cemento-enamel junction to the most apical extension of the gingival margin[3, 16-21]. Its aetiology includes factors:

- Anatomical - fenestration or dehiscence of the alveolar bone [18, 20, 22], poor tooth positioning[11, 20], aberrant tooth eruption pathway[20], individual tooth morphology[20, 23], shallow vestibule[2, 14, 17, 18, 20, 23, 24], muscle insertions near the gingival margin[14, 20, 22-25], thin keratinised gingiva[4, 18, 22, 26], inadequate alveolar bone crest thickness[24], root prominences[2, 13, 16, 20, 24];

- Pathological - periodontal disease [17, 18, 20, 25-30], dental caries[9, 14, 20], abrasion lesions[9, 16, 20], viral infection[30];

- Iatrogenic - orthodontic movement[4, 17, 18, 20, 22], inadequate restorations[9, 12, 18, 22, 24, 25, 27, 31], crowns with infragingival margins[27], smoking[7, 20, 32], lip/lingual piercing [24, 25];

- Mechanical - incorrect brushing[16, 18, 20, 22, 24, 33], occlusal trauma[18, 20, 22], surgical procedures[20].

Patients suffering from gingival recession most frequently complain of dental hypersensitivity and poor aesthetics[2, 7, 17, 18, 26]. Before considering surgical or non-surgical forms of periodontal therapy for the treatment of gingival recession' it is imperative to identify the aetiology of the problem[19]. One form of treatment for gingival recession is periodontal plastic surgery[21]. Miller defines this treatment as surgical procedures performed to correct or eliminate anatomical' developmental or traumatic deformities of the gingiva or alveolar mucosa' with root coverage surgery being the main component of this area[31]. Currently' there are several surgical techniques for this treatment:

- Pedicled soft tissue graft - advanced and rotational flap[12, 14, 19, 21, 24, 34-40];
- Free soft tissue graft - free gingival graft and connective tissue graft[9, 12, 21, 24, 31, 37, 40-45];

- Guided tissue regeneration with membranes[12, 21, 24, 40, 42, 43, 46, 47].

The main clinical indications for surgical treatment are: exposed roots; elongated clinical crowns and asymmetrical gingival margins that do not meet the patient's aesthetic requirements; absence of a minimum of keratinised gingiva (particularly when subgingival restorations or orthodontic treatment are planned); root hypersensitivity; predisposition to root caries; progressive gingival recessions[18]. The prognosis and success of root coverage surgery depend on several factors. Miller presented a classification of the various stages of gingival recession and their expected root coverage prognosis, taking into account the initial situation of apical migration of the gingival margin and interproximal bone loss:

- Class I: marginal gingival recession that does not extend to the mucogingival junction, without interproximal bone/tissue loss and in which 100 per cent root coverage is expected;
- Class II: marginal gingival recession that extends to or beyond the mucogingival junction, without interproximal bone/tissue loss and in which 100 per cent root coverage is expected;
- Class III: marginal gingival recession that extends to or beyond the mucogingival junction, with interproximal bone/tissue loss or tooth malposition and in which partial root coverage is expected;
- Class IV: marginal gingival recession extending to or beyond the mucogingival junction, with interproximal bone loss and/or tooth malposition so severe that root coverage cannot be anticipated. [11]

Miller suggested that periodontal plastic surgery for root coverage should provide a shallow sulcus and no bleeding after probing. Nevertheless, in general, the major advantages of this procedure for patients are the restoration of dental aesthetics and the reduction of tooth sensitivity[48]. The definition of complete root coverage, in which the procedure is considered successful, implies that the marginal soft tissue margin is located at the cemento-enamel junction, there is clinical adherence to the root, the sulcus depth is no more than two millimetres and there is no bleeding on probing. However, the first person to judge the success of the surgery is the patient and not the dentist[12, 41].

Currently, the scientific literature presents us with a relatively variable set of risk and success factors for this periodontal surgical therapy, accepted by most dentists. The aim of this bibliographical review is to survey those parameters that the scientific evidence states are or are not determining factors in the clinical outcome of root coverage surgery, to find the reasons for their classification in a particular category and to critically analyse them.

CHAPTER 2

MATERIALS AND METHODS

The aim of this monograph was to carry out a bibliographical review of the scientific literature by researching and analysing articles published in indexed journals (Portuguese/English), online and in print.

The bibliographic research for this study was carried out using the Natural Library of Medicine's electronic database PubMed-Medline and printed journals and periodontology textbooks available in the library of the Faculty of Dental Medicine of the University of Porto. For this purpose, a combination of the following keywords was sought: gingival recession; root coverage; periodontal disease; mucogingival defect; mucogingival surgery; periodontal plastic surgery.

The articles that were excluded during the literature search included studies with results obtained on animals, in vitro studies and articles with incomplete abstracts or unavailable full text.

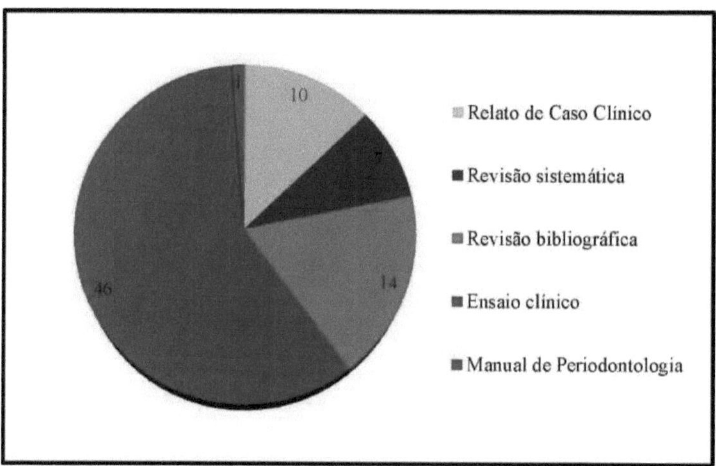

Graph I - Collected scientific articles grouped by category

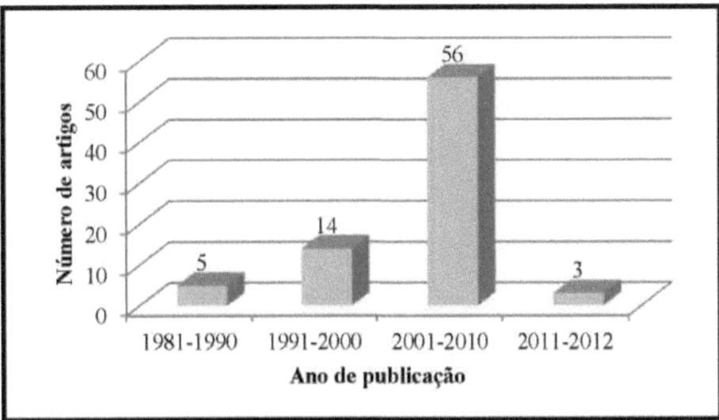

Graph II - Number of scientific articles included in the bibliographical research published per year

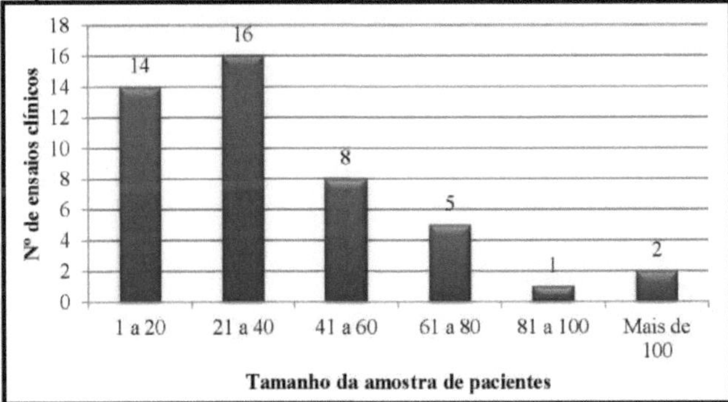

Graph III - Size of patient samples in clinical trial studies

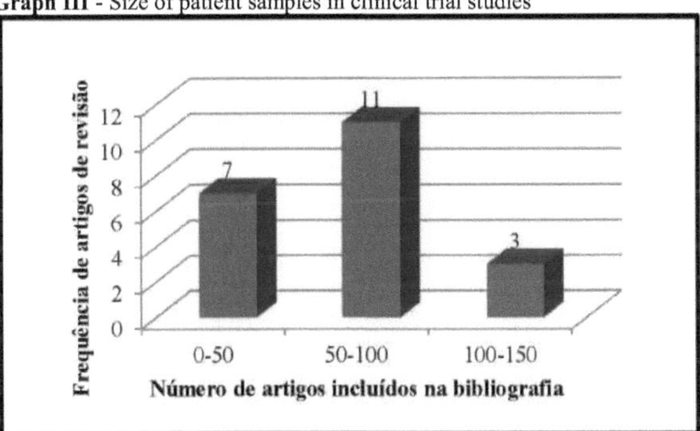

Graph IV - Number of scientific articles included in the bibliography of literature review and systematic review articles

CHAPTER 3

DISCUSSION

POST-PROBE HAEMORRHAGE

The presence of inflammation in the marginal gingiva is a criterion for assessing periodontal health, and is usually recorded through the assessment of periodontal probing, according to the principles of the Gingival Index (GI) or Post-Probing Haemorrhage (PPH), which has gradually replaced the first index in epidemiological studies[5] .

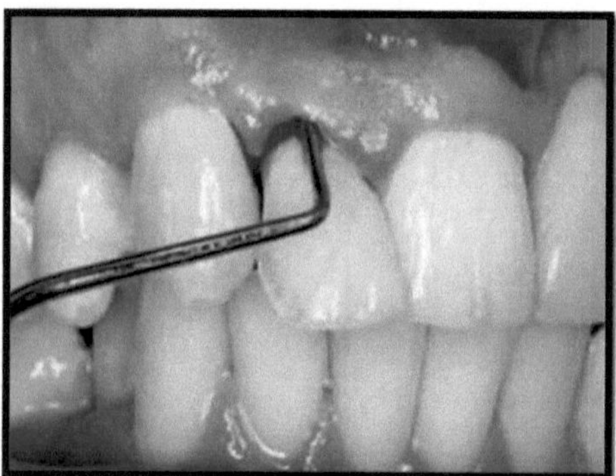

Figure I: probing the periodontal pocket of a lateral incisor, showing gingival haemorrhage after probing. [1]

Most scientific studies recommend that one of the requirements for achieving complete treatment success is for the patient to have an SPH index of less than 20-25% and no SPH in the sites that will undergo gingival surgery[2, 6, 26, 32, 34-37, 39, 49-51] , since the absence of bleeding after probing is an indicator of periodontal stability[1] . However, this parameter is not always an exclusion criterion, as all patients included in scientific studies have to go through a hygienic phase of improving and controlling their periodontal health, carried out by the dentist in their office and/or by the patient at home [2, 6, 7, 9, 20, 25, 26, 28-30, 32, 34, 36, 38, 39, 43, 45-47, 49, 50, 52-56]. In many situations, it is seen as a comparative parameter to assess the effectiveness of the hygienisation phase in controlling plaque and the outcome of surgical treatment in terms of periodontal health[7, 20, 23, 29, 32, 37, 38, 42-47, 49, 52, 53, 56] . In fact, the absence of bleeding after probing is one of the criteria presented by Miller as an indicator of success in complete root coverage[41] .

<u>**DENTAL PLAQUE**</u>

Dental plaque as a naturally occurring microbial deposit represents a biofilm, i.e. a relatively undefined microbial community associated with the tooth surface, in which the bacteria are in a matrix composed mainly of extracellular polymers of bacterial origin and products of gingival exudate and/or saliva[5] .

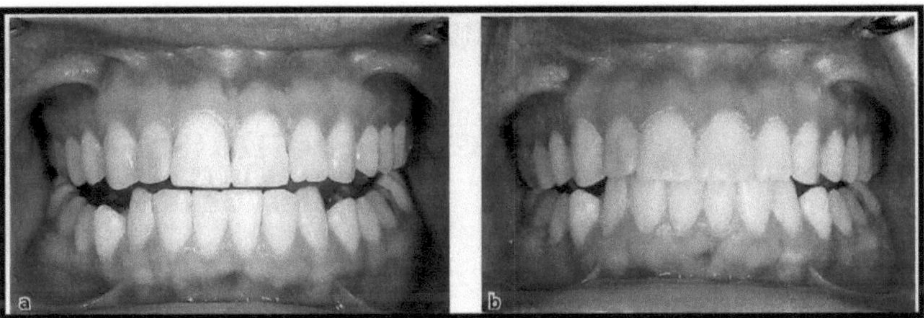

Figure II: experimental gingivitis model. **IIa:** A volunteer patient with clean teeth and clinically healthy gingival tissues at the start of the experimental period of plaque accumulation. **IIb:** The same patient 21 days after suspension of oral hygiene procedures, showing plaque deposits covering almost all tooth surfaces and consequently developing generalised inflammation in the marginal gingiva. [5]

Exposure of periodontal tissues to biofilm results in tissue inflammation, due to the interaction between bacterial infection and the host's immune response. Initially, the inflammation is restricted to the gums - gingivitis. With the maintenance of the etiological factors of inflammation, which can be dental plaque or secondary factors that promote its accumulation, the inflammatory response can evolve to the supporting periodontal tissues (bone and periodontal ligament), causing degradation of the matrix, resorption of the bone and apical migration of the epithelium - periodontitis[5, 18] .

Patients with poor oral hygiene and periodontal destruction have a higher risk of surgical failure, unless the local factors causing this poor hygiene can be controlled

oral[17] . Before any surgical periodontal treatment, the patient undergoes a hygiene phase, with oral hygiene instructions for their daily practice and oral hygiene appointments with the dentist, in order to comply with the standard requirement that the Plaque Index be less than 15-25% and that there be no bacterial plaque on the tooth surfaces to be submitted to surgery (2, 6, 7, 9, 10, 14, 16, 23, 25, 26, 28, 29, 32, 34-39, 42-47, 49-57). Notwithstanding this control, during the surgical procedure, the affected root surface is instrumented and smoothed to minimise the local inflammatory reaction and promote optimal healing of the surgical wound and favourable regeneration of the periodontal tissues (2, 7, 9, 10, 13-15, 20, 23, 25, 26, 28-32, 34-39, 41-47, 49-56, 58-68).

Miller (1985) states that complete root coverage can be expected in classes I and II, i.e. when there is no bone or interproximal tissue loss in the area affected by gingival recession. In classes III and IV, the greater the degree of interproximal bone and tissue loss or tooth malposition, the more difficult it is to predict the percentage of root coverage that can be achieved[11].

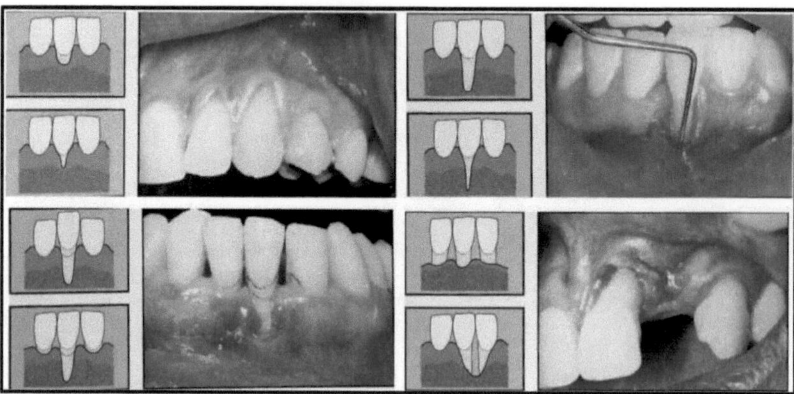

Figure III: Stages of gingival recession according to Miller's classification (I, II, III, IV), ordered sequentially from left to right, top to bottom. [11]

Although most of the scientific evidence is based on clinical studies carried out on Miller class I and II teeth, this factor is not an exclusion criterion. Rather, it seems to be due to the fact that it is possible to obtain more reliable results when assessing the effectiveness and limitations of a procedure and when comparing two or more procedures with each other, since in Miller classes I and II it is more likely to achieve complete root coverage[2, 6, 7, 14, 16, 23, 26, 29, 32, 36-38, 42-47, 49, 50, 53, 55]. In fact, there is also scientific evidence of clinical cases in which periodontal plastic surgery has been accepted for teeth in Miller classes III and IV, and in some cases it has been shown to be possible to achieve complete root coverage[20, 28, 51, 52, 54, 56, 57, 69].

HEIGHT OF GINGIVAL RECESSION

The height or depth of gingival recession is a parameter defined by the distance between the cemento-enamel junction and the most apical point of the gingival margin[6].

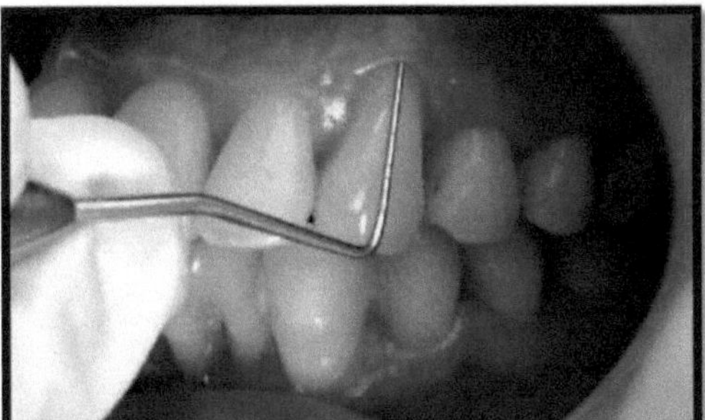

Figure IV: measuring the height of the gingival recession with a periodontal probe (6)

The likelihood of achieving complete root coverage decreases dramatically as the initial depth of the recession increases[70] . The greater the recession, the more difficult it is to move the gingival margin of the flap coronally to the cemento-enamel junction in the passive adaptation of the flap, which is the intended goal .[35]

However, this factor is not very relevant in the decision to carry out periodontal surgical therapy, but rather in the choice of surgical technique. Simple flap techniques are recommended for shallow recessions, while soft tissue grafting techniques and guided tissue regeneration are more suitable for very deep recessions[18] .

Regarding the admission of patients to the studies, the authors state that an initial depth of recession of more than two or three millimetres is necessary, as this parameter is used to assess the efficacy of the surgical technique studied or to compare the various techniques in the study (2, 6, 7, 32, 34, 35, 37, 43, 45, 46, 49, 53, 55, 56).

WIDTH OF GINGIVAL RECESSION

The width of the gingival recession is measured by the distance between the mesial and distal margins of the marginal gingiva, by placing a horizontally orientated probe on the most apical convexity of the cemento-enamel junction[14, 26, 42, 57] .

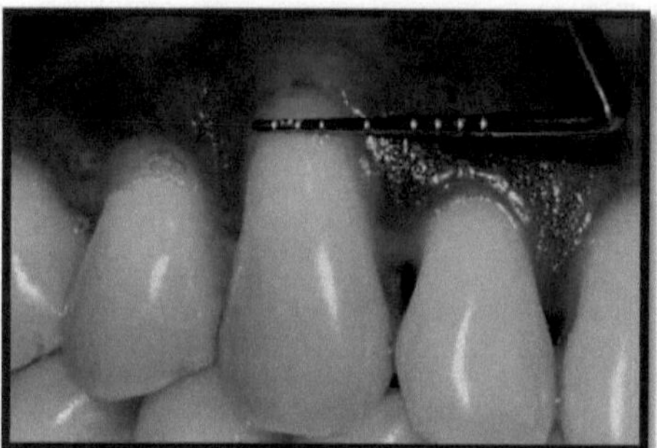

Figure V: measuring the width of the gingival recession with a periodontal probe. [14]

According to Sullivan and Atkins (1968), the most difficult type of recession to treat is one that is both deep (greater than or equal to 5 mm) and wide (greater than 3 mm), because it is too wide for a two-point collateral circulation to predictably cover the avascular zone[2, 58] .

For wide recessions, scientific evidence shows that connective tissue grafting is the most suitable technique for promoting complete root coverage, meeting the aesthetic needs of the patient and the requirements of the dentist[31] .

However, the width of the recession is a less strong predictor of the final result of periodontal surgery than the height of the recession, in terms of tissue healing. For this reason, there is no reference value for this parameter in terms of the likelihood of achieving complete root coverage[71] .

TOOTH VITALITY

Scientific evidence reports that non-vital teeth are rarely subjected to root coverage therapy studies[2, 6, 26, 28, 34-36, 43, 49, 50, 52, 56, 69] , so there are few studies on periodontal surgery associated with these teeth[28] . Korman and Robertson (2000) proved that endodontically treated teeth can respond differently to periodontal therapy. Sanders et al. (1983) confirmed this finding with a human study in which endodontically treated teeth responded less well to bone grafting to treat intraosseous defects[52] .

The interaction between the pulp and the periodontium and its effects on surgical wound healing have not yet been fully elucidated. There is some controversy as to the regenerative potential of adherence to the dentin surface of an endodontically treated tooth, although it has been documented that new conjunctival adherence can be formed to the cementum of non-vital teeth. The studies by Bjorn (1961, 1965), Diem (1974) and Mitsis (1970) revealed that radically endodontically treated teeth should respond to periodontal surgical therapy in the same way as vital teeth. Dunlap et al. (1981) reported that instrumented root surfaces of radically endodontically treated teeth were compatible with fibroblast growth in vitro[28] .

Vandana (2003) conducted a clinical study on root coverage surgery in vital and non-vital teeth, where he demonstrated that the reduction in probing depth, the gain in clinical adherence level and the filling of the bone defect and its resolution were seen in both vital and non-vital teeth[28] .

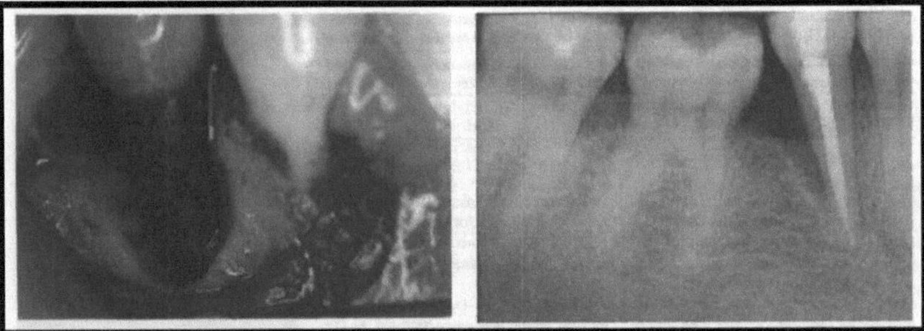

Figure VI: Deep distal intraosseous defect and buccal dehiscence affecting a lower second premolar (left); initial radiograph showing the defect and root canal filling, with no associated periapical radiolucency (right). [52]

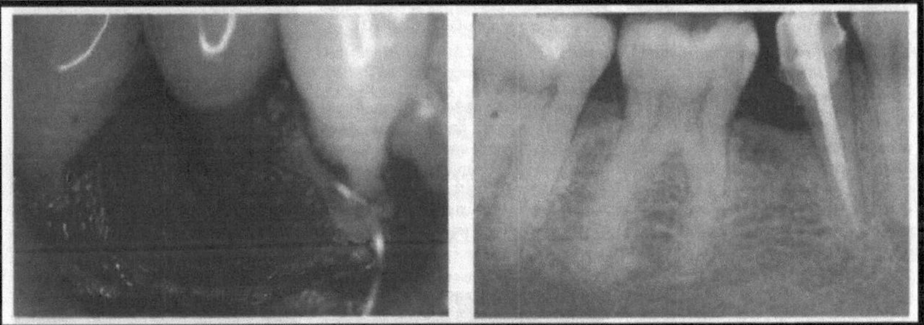

Figure VII: bioabsorbable membrane positioned to cover the defect (left); radiograph one year after surgery, showing complete resolution of the intraosseous component of the defect (right). [52]

<u>GINGIVAL DIMENSIONS</u>

One of the indications for root coverage surgery is inadequate gingival width[17, 22, 24, 26] . The dimensions of the gingiva influence the occurrence of gingival recession, the choice of surgical technique and the prognosis of root coverage[40, 72] , and there is a negative correlation between the average width of attached gingiva and the number of gingival recessions .[33]

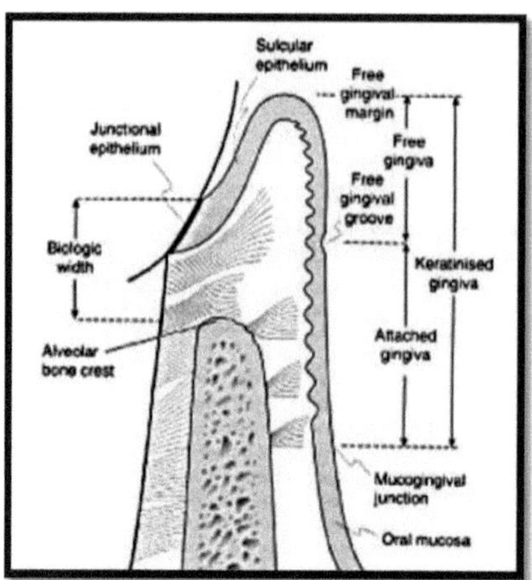

Figure VIII: anatomy of the gingiva. The gingiva can be divided into keratinised and non-keratinised, which are separated by the mucogingival junction. Keratinised gingiva is made up of adhered gingiva and free gingiva (4).

It is believed that the prevalence of gingival recessions increases significantly when the thickness of keratinised gingiva is less than 2 mm, the reference value for good gingival health, which suggests that periodontal surgery is more likely to be successful when the dimensions of attached gingiva are equal to or greater than this value[7, 33] . To overcome this problem, laterally repositioned flaps, double papilla flaps, soft tissue grafts and guided tissue regeneration are techniques indicated when gingival dimensions are insufficient to provide complete root coverage .[65]

The thickness of the gingiva has direct implications for the healing of the surgical wound, flap maintenance, the intensity of gingival inflammation, orthodontic treatment decisions, the propensity to develop gingival recession and the choice of flap type[4] .

The size of the attached gingiva depends on the height of the alveolar process and the size of the lower face, and is generally greater in men. With regard to facial attached gingiva, the thickness is usually greater in the maxilla than in the mandible. The thinnest thickness is found in the maxillary canine and mandibular first premolar, at 0.7-0.9 mm; in the central and lateral incisors, it is slightly below 3 mm; in the second premolar and second molar, it is slightly above 3 mm; the greatest thickness is found in the third molar, estimated to be around 4 mm[4, 33] .

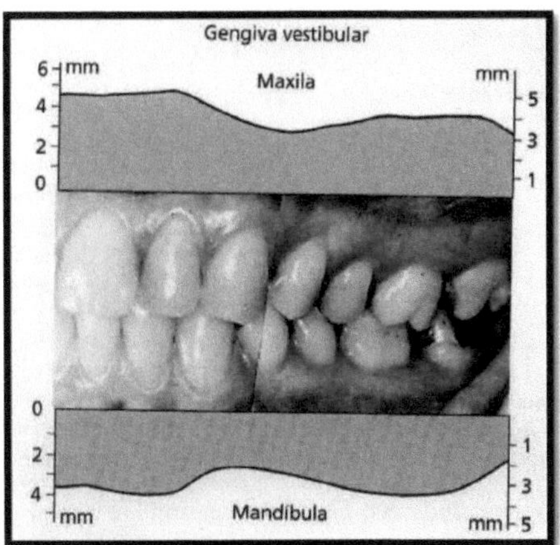

Figure IX: Variation in the width of the adhered gingiva on the different maxillary and mandibular teeth. (5)

According to the aforementioned gingival thickness values, canines and first pre-molars are the teeth most frequently affected by gingival recessions. However, the frequency of gingival recessions is not significantly different between left and right maxillary canines and first pre-molars, and is only slightly different between right and left mandibular canines and first pre-molars. This is expected to be caused by brushing trauma depending on the directing hand[33] .

Maxillary teeth are more likely to undergo gingival augmentation through periodontal plastic surgery than mandibular teeth, which is certainly due to the downward direction of blood microcirculation in the upper arch compared to the upward direction in the lower arch. The greater the loss of adherence related to gingival recession, the greater the need for gingival augmentation[69] . Not limited to the presence of gingival recessions, gingival augmentation can be advantageous in areas with subgingival restorations or deep cervical abrasions, precisely to prevent this problem .[12]

Zuchelli and de Sanctis (2007) showed that the increase in keratinised gingiva in root coverage surgery was more significant in sites with a greater depth of recession and a lower initial amount of keratinised gingiva[14] .

In this chapter, the dimensions of the interdental papilla should also be emphasised in the prognosis of root coverage, namely its diameter, height and thickness.[14, 50, 55] . Loss of height of the interdental papilla can limit root coverage, as it reduces the potential advancement of the coronal flap and reduces vascular exchange between the soft tissues covering the root and the interdental connective tissue[3] . Saletta et al. (2001) found that root coverage is not significantly correlated with the area or height of the interdental papilla, but is significantly more frequent in sites with lower interdental papilla height[50] . Bouchard et al. (2000) report that the loss of the interdental papilla can be partially resolved

17

in isolated defects by grafting .[12, 22]

ORAL HYGIENE

An incorrect or traumatic brushing technique, neglect in maintaining good oral hygiene and the use of improper oral hygiene techniques (using a toothpick or fingernails) are etiological factors of gingival recession and, at the same time, risk factors for the failure of root coverage surgery[7, 16-18, 20, 22, 24, 29, 33, 45, 57, 71] . In fact, loss of adherence and gingival recession are predominantly found on the oral surfaces of teeth in populations that maintain a high level of oral hygiene .[29]

An altered brushing technique is of greater significance for the long-term result of root coverage than gingival dimensions. Khocht et al. (1993) revealed in their study that gingival recession is associated with the use of hard brushes: all the patients included in the study used some kind of modification of the Bass technique or another non-specific technique, which created apically directed pressure on the marginal soft tissue[29] .

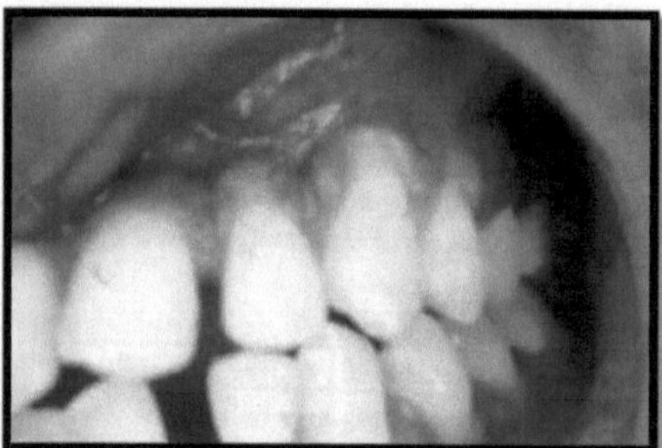

Figure X: gingival recession associated with traumatic tooth brushing. [21]

SMOKING

Smoking is one of the factors most associated with the incidence of gingival recession, and this strong association seems to be independent of the severity of interproximal attachment loss and dependent on the level of exposure to tobacco, although the latter association is still a matter of controversy among authors[32, 69] . It has also been identified as a detrimental agent for the short- and long-term results of periodontal surgery procedures. Therefore, the patient's smoking status should be carefully assessed if their treatment plan includes surgical correction of gingival recession .[24, 69, 71]

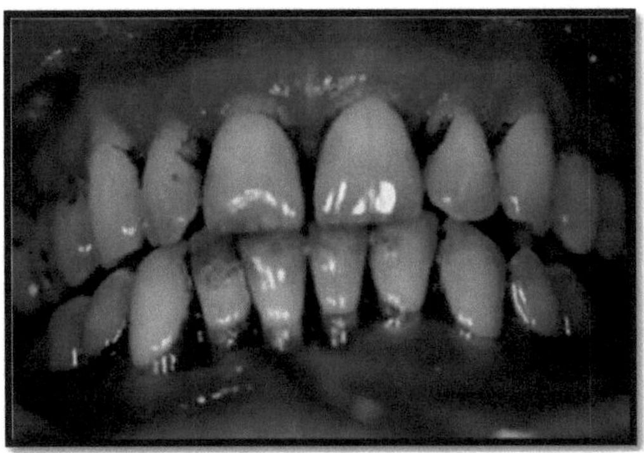

Figure XI: Tooth pigmentation, gingival recession, alveolar bone loss and periodontal pockets resulting from the deteriorative effect of smoking habits (7).

Smoking has a primary systemic influence by altering the host response and/or damaging periodontal cells. Nicotine has been shown in vitro to affect fibroblast proliferation, increase collagenase activity and inhibit fibroblast synthesis of fibronectin and type I collagen. Insufficient oxygen transport and metabolism caused by carbon monoxide, as well as enzymatic poisoning caused by hydrogen cyanide, reduce the oxidative metabolism necessary for cell repair to occur[7] . In this sense, clinical studies recommend that patients who are going to undergo periodontal surgery should not be smokers or should be willing to quit smoking[26, 32, 43, 44, 47, 49, 53, 54, 58] , since smoking causes periodontal destruction and hinders healing after surgery, leading to worse results in periodontal therapy .[17, 32]

Specifically, it is known that active smoking counteracts the gain in clinical adherence[71] . Martins et al. (2004) compared the effects of smoking on the outcome of root coverage surgery in smokers and non-smokers, finding that smokers had a lower percentage of root coverage, less gain in clinical adherence and greater probing depth compared to non-smokers .[7]

TOOTH MORPHOLOGY

Gingival height, thickness and contours are parameters that can vary considerably in a population, which translates into different gingival phenotypes. The symptoms of periodontal disease, namely gingival recession and increased probing depths, can vary depending on the periodontal phenotype. Therefore, the morphological characteristics of the periodontium may be related to dental anatomy[26] .

Olsson and Lindhe (1991) studied the periodontal characteristics of individuals with varying maxillary central incisor shapes and found that there were two types of crowns: long and thin crowns and short and wide crowns. They concluded that the prevalence of gingival recession is higher in patients with maxillary incisors with long, thin crowns[26] .

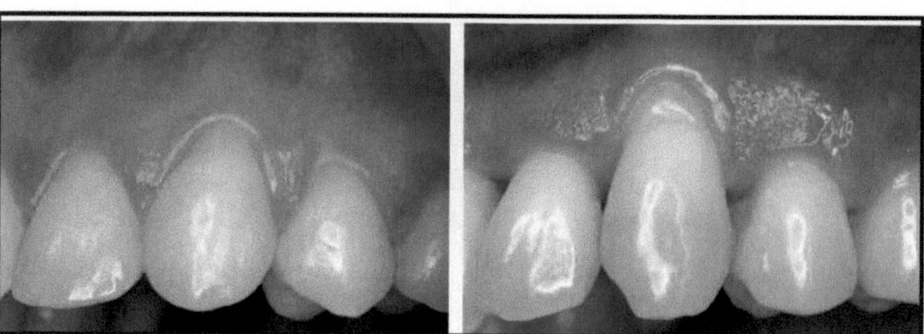

Figure XII: types of dental crowns according to Olsson and Lindhe (1991). On the left, a short, wide crown; on the right, a long, thin crown. [26]

In terms of surgical periodontal therapy, there are no studies showing the influence of the shape of the tooth crown on the outcome of root coverage surgery. Peres et al. (2009) sought to test this link and found that there is an influence of crown shape on the morphology of the periodontium, but that this association does not affect the final outcome of the surgery[26] .

With regard to the shape of the tooth, there are three factors of great importance in the success of root coverage surgery: absence of irregularities or grooves in the root[2, 35, 36] ; slight convexity of the root; absence of root prominences[2, 16, 65] .

Holbrook and Ochsenbein (1983) suggested that during root coverage surgery, vigorous root smoothing should be performed to eliminate irregularities and grooves, reduce root convexity and thus decrease the mesio-distal distance between the periodontal spaces[2] . However, the extent of the reduction in root prominence is empirical[13] .

Anatomically, the most difficult exposed root surface to cover is the root of the maxillary canine. As it is located at the corner of the dental arch, it has a pronounced mesio-distal curvature, has pronounced mesio-distal and occluso-apical convexities and concavities are present mesial and distal to the root prominence. Root straightening produces a considerable reduction in cementum thickness. The convexity of the root is diminished and therefore this theoretically minimises the mesio-distal dimension of the surface[13] .

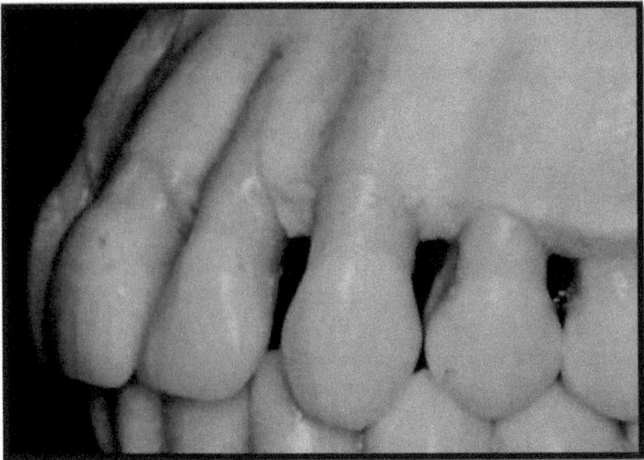

Figure XIII: profile view of the maxillary arch of a dry skull. Fenestrations and dehiscences are obvious. Different curvatures are visible between the roots of the various teeth. [13]

MUSCLE INSERTIONS

The presence of bridles and other aberrant muscle insertions close to the gingival margin is an etiological factor in gingival recession[14, 18, 20, 23-25] , as well as a limitation in the choice of surgical technique[23] .

Stretching the gingiva in its facial aspect, resulting in a reduced buccolingual dimension of marginal tissue, can favour the destructive effect of inflammatory lesions associated with plaque[22] . Therefore, in order to maximise the adaptation of the flap to the tooth, the scientific literature recommends, before or during root coverage surgery, eliminating the muscle insertions included in the thickness of the flap, which eliminates labial tension on the flap and passively positions it in a coronal position[14]

.

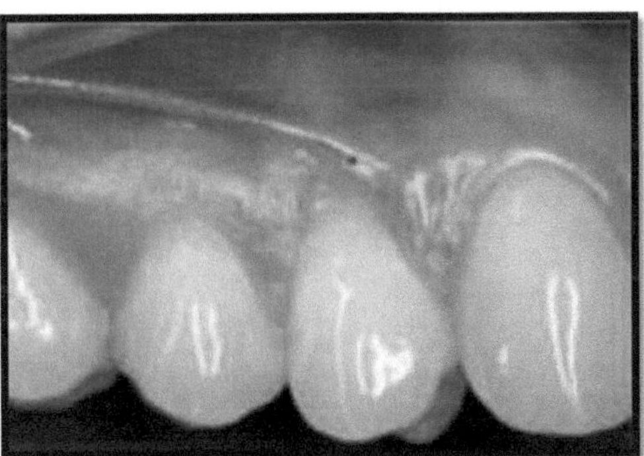

Figure XV: Exposed root with non-carious lesion in the maxillary first premolar. Note the high insertion of the labial brake.[12]

THICKNESS, TENSION AND ADAPTATION OF THE SOFT TISSUE FLAP

Wound healing after mucogingival surgery depends on coagulation, revascularisation and maintenance of blood supply[12, 73] . In root coverage surgery, flap survival depends on the degree of primary and collateral blood supply. Full thickness flaps preserve vascular patency and show dilation of the supraperiosteal blood vessels; if there is adequate tissue adaptation, revascularisation between the flap and the underlying bone is established within a few days; as the flap vasculature is preserved intact, the surgical wound normally heals, regardless of anatomical variations in blood supply in each individual. On the other hand, partial thickness flaps preserve fewer intact gingival blood vessels, depending largely on the compensatory blood circulation of the bone and periodontal ligament[73] . However, flap thickness has only become a common clinical measurement more recently, and there is not enough scientific evidence to assess its influence on periodontal surgery[40, 53, 55, 58] . Hwang and Wang (2006) studied flap thickness as a predictor of root coverage and were unable to elucidate its effect according to the various surgical techniques used, which indicates the need for more controlled clinical trials on this subject[73] . Baldi and Pini Prato (1999, 2000) pointed out the importance of flap thickness and tension in the clinical results of coronally positioned flaps[50] . Esteibar et al. (2011) concluded that one of the important factors for achieving success in periodontal surgery is the presence of a flap with a thickness of more than 2 mm[58] . Another factor that is relevant to the outcome of mucogingival surgery is the tension of the flap before it is sutured[2, 14, 40, 50, 55, 56] . It is known that recurrent recessions can be associated with high flap tension, so flap displacement requires flap relaxation and passive adaptation without tension at the cemento-enamel junction .[2]

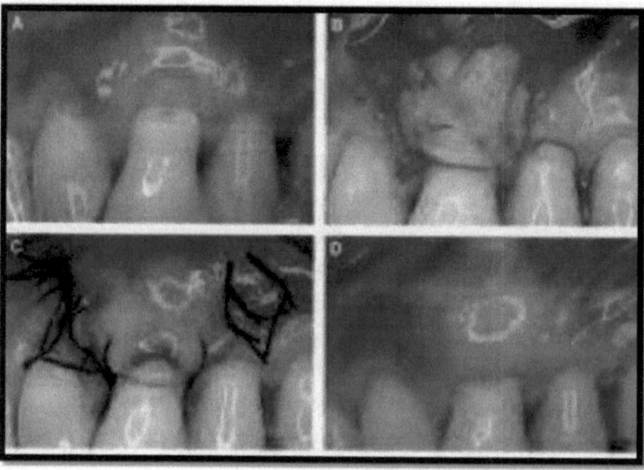

Figure XIV: Coronally repositioned flap with connective tissue graft, applied to a gingival recession associated with an abrasion lesion. Note the passive adaptation of the flap, without tension. (8)

<u>POST-SURGICAL POSITION OF THE GINGIVAL MARGIN</u>

One of the criteria that is considered indispensable for successful root coverage is that the gingival margin is located at the cemento-enamel junction. There is a causal relationship between the gingival margin and complete root coverage: the greater the height of the recession, the more difficult it is to move the gingival margin of the flap coronally to the cemento-enamel junction in the passive adaptation of the flap[35] .

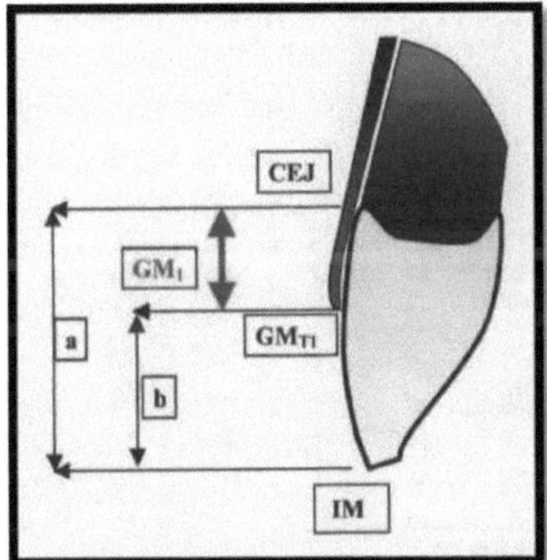

Figure XVI: calculation of the location of the gingival margin after suturing (GM1) respecting the enamel-cement junction **(CEJ)**. [2]
GM1 = a - b = IMCEJ - IMGMT1.
IM = incisal margin;
GMᴛɪ = gingival margin after suturing;
a = distance between **IM** and **CEJ**;
b = distance between **IM** and GMᴛ1;
GM1 = distance between the gingival margin and the enamel-cement junction immediately after surgery, calculated as **a - b**.

After root coverage surgery, a phenomenon called creeping attachment occurs in the flap, which consists of the postoperative migration of the gingival margin in a coronal direction of a previously denuded root[58] . Contraction of the surgical wound is a major event that occurs during the formation of granulation tissue[12] . It is not predictable, is generally reported in recessions less than 3 mm wide and is best observed in anterior mandibular teeth, and can be detected one to twelve months after surgery .[15]

Pini Prato et al. (2005) studied the relationship between the post-surgical position of the gingival margin and the frequency of complete root coverage. They found that few cases in which the gingival margin was positioned at the cemento-enamel junction resulted in complete root coverage, while all cases in which the gingival margin was positioned 2 mm coronally to the cemento-enamel junction achieved complete root coverage. They concluded that it is prudent to suture the gingival margin at least 2 mm coronally to the cemento-enamel junction in order to achieve complete root coverage, because the more coronal the gingival margin is after suturing, the greater the likelihood of complete root coverage[2] .

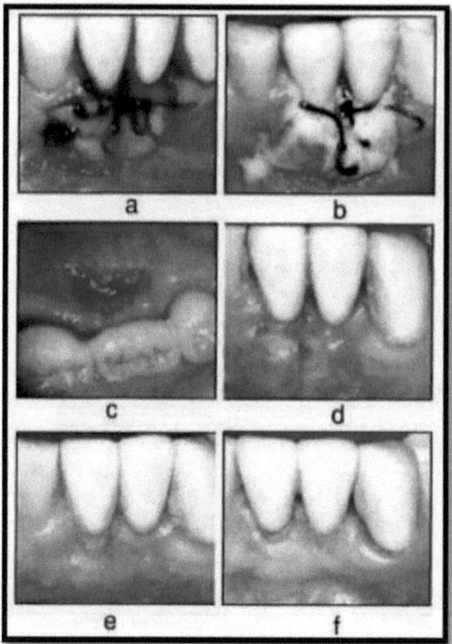

Figure XVII: (a) Stabilisation of the flap at the recipient site with interrupted and crossed sutures. (b) Partial necrosis of the flap evident one week after surgery. (c) Secondary healing of the donor site surgical wound one week after surgery. (d) Oedematous phase of graft healing two weeks after surgery. (e) Six weeks after surgery, an increased amount of firm gingival tissue apically and partial root coverage of the exposed root via the bridging mechanism. (f) Considerable increase in the amount of firm gingival tissue as well as an increased amount of root coverage by *creeping attachment* are evident one year after connective tissue graft surgery on tooth #31.[15]

The most frequent error in the selection of reference parameters is the location of the anatomical cemento-enamel junction. In many situations, cervical lesions involve the crown and exposed root, causing the anatomical cemento-enamel junction to disappear[9] . Furthermore, in many cases of gingival recessions associated with cervical abrasion, a line appears separating the enamel from the coronal dentin, which is often mistaken for the cemento-enamel junction .[3]

The predictability of root coverage of a given surgical procedure is assessed in terms of the percentage of root coverage and the percentage of surfaces with complete root coverage. When the cemento-enamel junction is not present, it is no longer possible to measure the depth and width of the recession or to assess the effectiveness of a surgical technique in terms of root coverage[3] . Therefore, the difficulty in identifying it is a major limitation and consequently an exclusion criterion for root coverage surgery[2, 16, 32, 34-36, 49, 50, 55] .

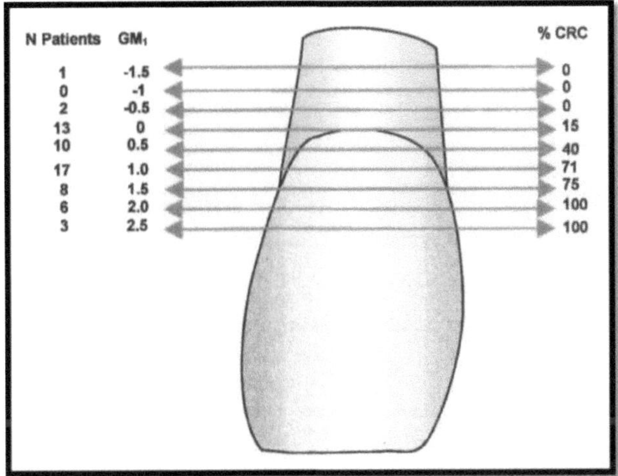

Figure XVIII: relationship between the location of the gingival margin, in mm, after suturing (GM1) and the frequency of complete root coverage (CRC).[3]

In order to overcome this impediment, Zucchelli et al. (2006) proposed a method of predetermining the clinical cemento-enamel junction, which can be used to assess the results of root coverage when the anatomical cemento-enamel junction is not observable, to improve the aesthetic result of root coverage surgery and to allow the combination of restorative and periodontal treatment of a cervical abrasion associated with gingival recession. This happens particularly in situations of loss of height of the interdental papilla, extrusion or rotation of the tooth, occlusal abrasion and cervical abrasion[3]

.

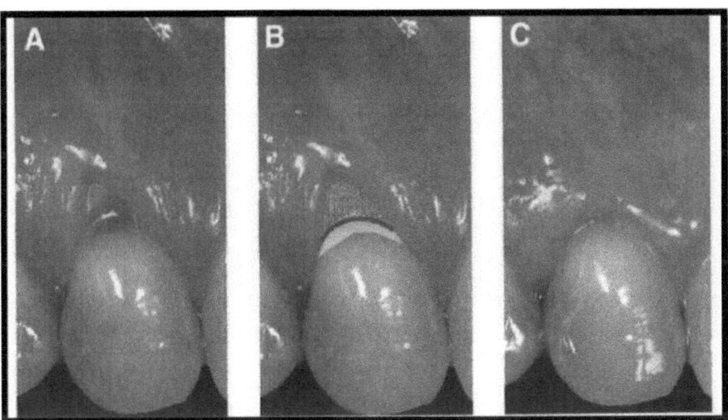

Figure XIX: Combined restorative-periodontal treatment of a cervical abrasion associated with gingival recession. **(A)** A canine with gingival recession and a deep abrasive defect. The anatomical cemento-enamel junction has disappeared. **(B)** The clinical cemento-enamel junction (red line) is located in the deepest part of the abrasive defect. The area of abrasion coronal to the cemento-enamel junction was restored with composite (white area), while the apical portion (shaded area) of the defect, along with root exposure, was treated with root coverage surgery. (C) 1-year follow-up after restoration with composite and root coverage surgery. The clinical crown length was reduced to predetermine the location of the clinical cemento-enamel junction.[3]

DIMENSIONS OF THE INTRAOSSEOUS DEFECT

The presence of an intraosseous defect and its height and width have a strong impact on the results of periodontal therapy. Vertical adhesion gain describes the bone and soft tissue components of periodontal healing[71] .

The mucogingival line has a tendency to recover its predefined position "genetically" after its coronal displacement. The possibility of achieving a new conjunctival attachment, in theory, should be considerably greater in short defects than in wide ones, probably because the periodontal ligament in the lateral parts of the defect serves as a source of granulation tissue from which a new attachment can develop[29] .

Cortellini et al. (1998) demonstrated that the linear amount of improvement in the results tested was greater in deep defects than in superficial defects and that the percentage gain in clinical adherence, taking into account the depth of the defect, was similar in superficial and deep defects. This led to the conclusion that the regeneration potential is similar in superficial and deep defects[51] .

Klein et al. (2001) found that the angle and depth of the intraosseous defect influence vertical adhesion gains, but that six months after periodontal surgery, the vertical adhesion gain in deep and shallow intraosseous defects was the same, and that guided tissue regeneration resulted in statistically more favourable bone filling in deep and short bone defects than in wide and shallow defects[71] .

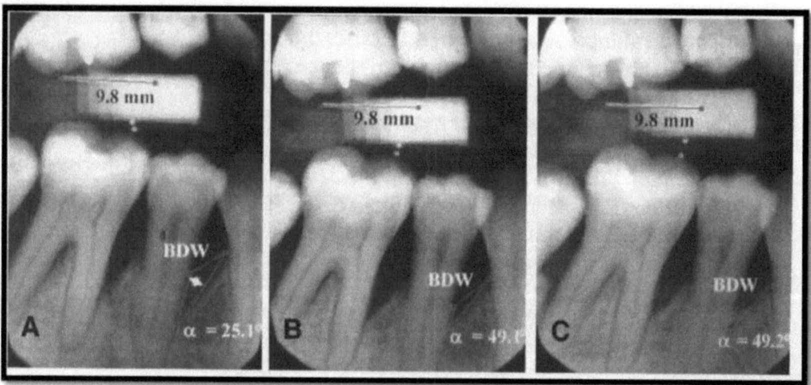

Figure XX: Mesial intraosseous defect of tooth #45. (**A**) Initial radiograph. (**B**) 6 months after root coverage surgery with guided tissue regeneration. (**C**) 24 months after surgery. [71]

VESTIBULE DEPTH

A shallow vestibule can be an etiological or aggravating factor in gingival recession and also a limitation in the choice of root coverage surgical technique[2, 14, 17, 18, 20, 24] . Pini Prato et al. (2005) indicated that the presence of a short vestibule may be associated with deep gingival recessions, since the forces caused by lip movements are transmitted more intensely to the facial gingiva, generating greater tension in the marginal gingiva .[2]

ORTHODONTIC MOVEMENT

When gingival dimensions are not taken into account when planning orthodontic treatment, orthodontic forces can induce the development of gingival recessions, although the presence of a certain amount of gingiva does not seem to be essential for maintaining periodontal health and preventing gingival recession[22] . There is some controversy as to whether periodontal treatment should be prioritised over orthodontic treatment and vice versa. However, if there is a malocclusion that is inducing the development of gingival recessions, orthodontic treatment must be considered with or without periodontal surgery .[20, 74]

When the tooth enters the oral cavity during eruption, the reduced enamel epithelium and the alveolar mucosal epithelium fuse at the top of the tooth. This means that there is no wounding of the connective tissue and, consequently, no granulation tissue is formed. Therefore, mucogingival problems such as gingival recessions will initially be eliminated spontaneously during growth, as long as adequate dental plaque control is ensured[22] .

Orthodontic treatment can create a situation that exposes teeth favourable to the development of recession defects: a thin or inadequate gingival zone is a reason to observe soft tissue recession in conjunction with orthodontic movement. However, orthodontic forces alone do not induce loss of conjunctival adhesion, and the integrity of the periodontium can be maintained during orthodontic treatment, even in areas with a minimal amount of gingiva. As long as the tooth moves exclusively within the alveolar bone, soft tissue recession cannot develop. A facially positioned tooth often shows dehiscence of the alveolar bone with thin soft tissue covering it, but when it is moved in a lingual direction to a more suitable position within the alveolar process, the dimensions of the tissue in its facial aspect will increase in thickness, which in turn results in an increased height of free gingiva and a decreased height of the clinical crown[22, 75, 76] .

The thickness, rather than the quality, of the marginal soft tissue on the pressure side of the tooth seems to be the determining factor for the development of recessions during orthodontic treatment in dentitions affected by bacterial plaque. The stretching of the facial gingiva, resulting in a reduced buccolingual dimension of marginal tissue, can favour the destructive effect of inflammatory lesions associated with bacterial plaque[22, 65] .

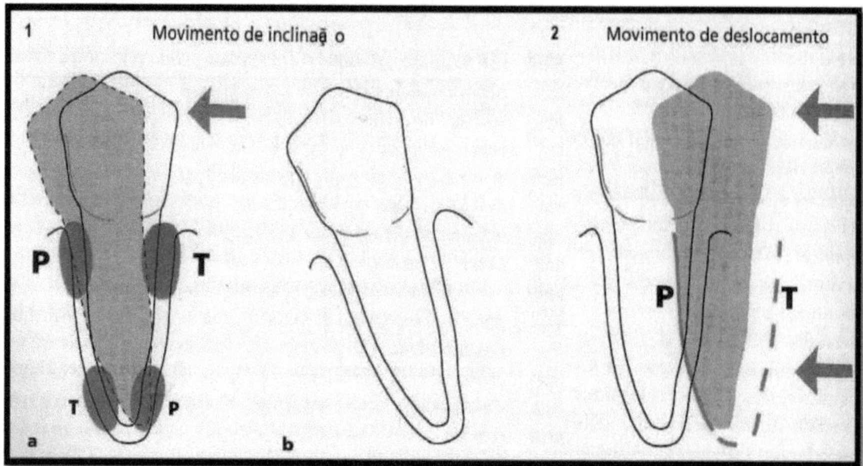

Figure XXI:

(1) If the tooth crown is subjected to excessive horizontally orientated forces (arrow), pressure (P) and tension (T) zones will appear in the marginal and apical areas of the periodontium (a). The supra-alveolar connective tissue is not affected by the application of force. In the pressure and tension zones, tissue changes occur which eventually allow the tooth to tilt in the direction of the force. When the tooth is no longer subjected to trauma, complete repair of the periodontal tissues occurs (b). There is no apical migration of the gingival epithelium.

(2) When the tooth is exposed to forces that produce "displacement", as in orthodontic treatment, the pressure (P) and tension (T) zones, depending on the direction of the force, extend to the entire surface of the tooth. The supra-alveolar connective tissue is not affected either in association with the tilting movement or the displacement movement. Forces of this type will therefore not cause inflammatory reactions in the gingiva. There is no apical migration of the gingival epithelium. [5]

CROWN AND RESTORATION MARGINS

The interaction between Periodontology, Dentistry and Fixed Prosthodontics is threefold, namely in the margins of the restoration, the contours of the crown and the response of the gingival tissues. Placing restoration or crown margins within the biological space often leads to gingival inflammation, loss of clinical adherence and bone loss, which is clinically manifested by deeper periodontal pockets or gingival recession. The closer the margin of a subgingival crown is to epithelial adhesion, the more likely it is that severe gingival inflammation will occur[3, 27] .

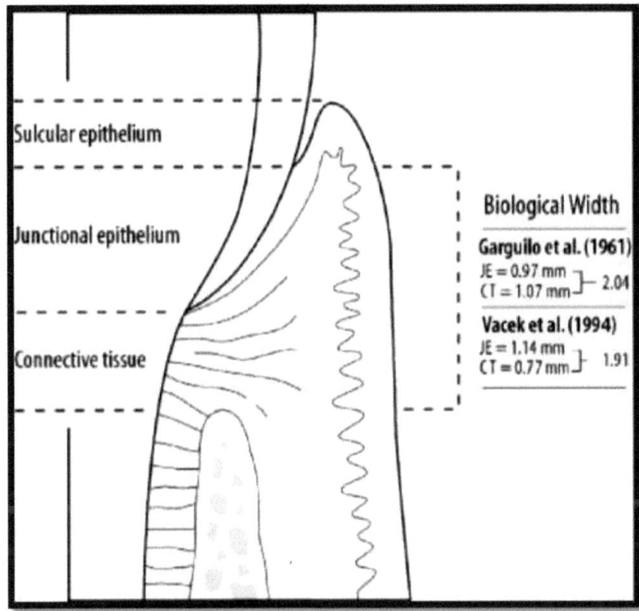

Figure XXII: biological space. [27]

The location of restorative margins is determined by various factors, including aesthetics, retentive factors, susceptibility to root caries and the degree of gingival recession. However, although crown margins can be placed subgingivally, it is very likely that over time they will become supragingival[27]

.

The patient's aesthetic demands often require the margins of the restoration or crown to be "buried", which can lead to a violation of the biological space. When preparation of subgingival margins is indicated, the dentist must avoid breaking the junction epithelium or conjunctival adhesion during preparation and impressions, and when the margins end at or near the level of the alveolar crest, surgical lengthening of the crown is necessary. It seems prudent to guarantee a minimum of 3 mm of space between the margins and the alveolar bone during treatment planning. In cases where an inadequate thickness of keratinised gingiva is observed, the dentist should consider performing a gingival augmentation on teeth with a minimum of keratinised gingiva before placing restorations with subgingival margins[12, 27] .

Subgingival margins show greater plaque accumulation, bleeding on probing, probing depth and are more associated with spirochetes, fusiform, wheel and filamentous bacteria. In fact, posterior teeth with crowns or proximal restorations are more frequently associated with furcation involvement and loss of clinical adherence than teeth without proximal restorations[25, 27] .

Pack et al. (1990) reported that periodontal disease is more severe when overflowing restorations are present, as they contribute to gingival inflammation due to their ability to retain bacterial plaque. In fact, overflowing restorations not only increase the amount of plaque, they also increase the presence of specific periodontal pathogens in the plaque, with changes in the associated bacterial microflora to that seen in adult chronic periodontitis. Most overflowing restorations can be recontoured without having to remove the restoration[9, 27] .

Some authors state that an artificial crown should follow the original anatomy of the tooth contour to allow functional stimulation and maintain gingival health, while others state that crowns should be sub-contoured to achieve better periodontal health[27] . The presence of loose or open proximal contacts contributes to the formation of periodontal pockets. Hancock et al. (1980) found a significant relationship between food impaction and the type of contact and between food impaction and probing depth. While the role of poor interproximal integrity appears to be unclear, open contacts that lead to food impaction are uncomfortable for the patient, and it is accepted that strong interproximal contacts are important for gingival health[27] .

Often, the mistake of not performing surgery before placing the margins in these situations leads to the margins being placed too close to the alveolar crest, thus invading the biological space. This can be achieved not only by surgical lengthening but also by orthodontic forced eruption or a combination of both. At least 3 mm of distance is needed between the bone crest and the margin of the final restoration after surgical lengthening of the crown, to allow the margin to end supragingivally. In teeth with an indication for crowns, the dentist must ensure sufficient coronal exposure to allow adequate retention of the crown, planning a distance of 4 mm from the margin of the restoration to the alveolar crest. In this way, the biological space is re-established after the procedure, the junctional epithelium is established in the apical portion of the root plan and space is created for the supracrestal connective tissue through crystal resorption of the alveolar bone[27] .

SUBGINGIVAL RESTORATIONS

Subgingival restorations are more likely to bleed and exhibit gingival recession than supragingival restorations, as they are plaque-retentive areas and are inaccessible to scraping and root planing instruments[27] . The presence of a restoration in the root does not preclude the possibility of root coverage, but theoretically it should be removed before the root is covered with soft tissue .[5]

In gingival recessions associated with deep caries or cervical abrasions, complete coverage by conventional mucogingival surgery techniques may be contraindicated due to the need for extensive root preparation that could compromise the tooth, particularly on root surfaces where cavity preparation and/or cervical abrasion exceeds a depth of 1-3 mm[2, 6, 26, 32, 34-36, 49, 53, 55, 58] . Procedures that move the soft tissues coronally into the abrasion regions can hinder the patient's plaque control and make the restorative procedure more difficult. In this sense, combining an adhesive restoration with a surgical overlay may be the solution[9] . The roughness and subgingival position of acrylic resin restorations have been shown to be key factors in the development of gingival inflammation. Furthermore, in a study in dogs, it was found that the inflammatory infiltrate associated with amalgam restorations was more intense than that associated with resin-modified glass ionomer restorations. Therefore, the use of adhesive restorative materials has proven to be a biocompatible alternative for restoring deep caries or cervical abrasions prior to surgical root coverage[9] .

Dragoo et al. (1997) observed that subgingival areas in patients with large root lesions restored with resin-modified glass ionomer had clinically healthy periodontal tissues that were well adapted to the root surface, with no bleeding on probing and minimal sulcus depth. Histologically, he found that fibroblasts and connective tissue adhered to the restorations. Subsequently, Alkan et al. (2006) noted the occurrence of creeping attachment in resin-modified glass ionomer restorations at monthly check-ups[9, 15] .

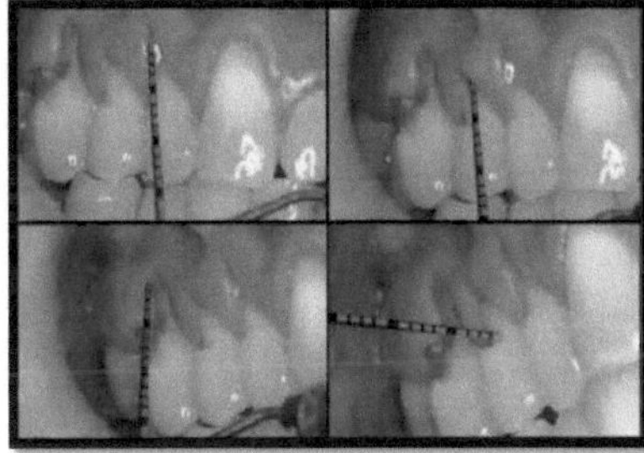
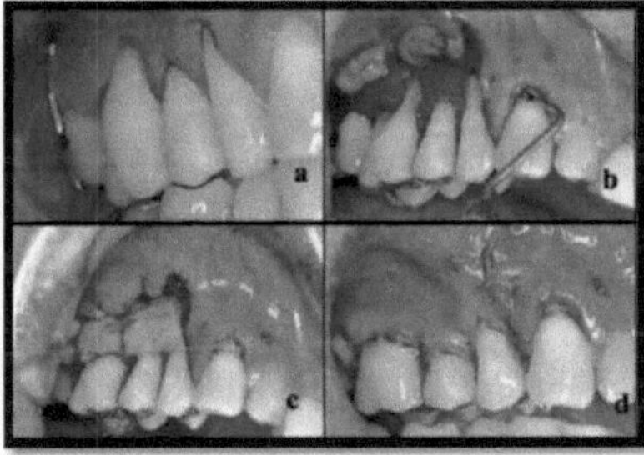

Figure XXIII: Pre-operative clinical photograph showing multiple and adjacent gingival recessions associated with deep cervical abrasions on teeth #14, #15 and #16, caused by brushing trauma. (9)
Figure XXIV: (a) Deep cervical abrasions restored with microparticulate composite resin; (b) Partial thickness flap reflected from the distal surface of tooth #13 to the mesial surface of tooth #17; (c) Subepithelial connective tissue graft positioned and sutured to the recipient site; (d) Coronal flap sutured. (9)

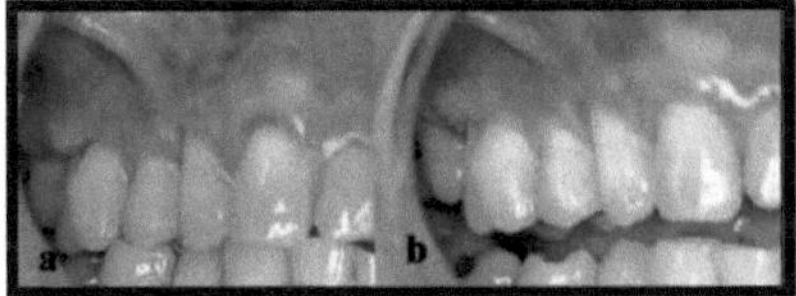

Figure XXV: Post-operative course. (a) 2 months; (b) 8 months.(9)

Martins et al. (2007) analysed the histological response of periodontal tissues to class V composite and resin-modified glass ionomer restorations and noted the biocompatibility of all the materials tested. However, adhesive restorations are always subject to physical challenges - occlusal masticatory forces, repetitive expansion, shrinkage stress due to thermal variations - and chemical challenges - dentin fluid, saliva, bacterial products, food, drink - over time. These factors act on the tooth/restoration interface and result in various patterns of degradation of collagen fibrils and resin components. Van Dijken and Sjòstròm (1998) found that areas restored with resin-modified glass ionomer cements and composites were associated with greater amounts of gingival crevicular fluid compared to unrestored areas[9, 27].

To circumvent the problems that subgingival restorations present to periodontal health, Camargo et al. (2001) state that intense plaque control using a correct brushing technique with non-excessive force is important for maintaining long-term health in areas undergoing root coverage associated with restorative procedures[9, 27, 77].

MALOCCLUSION

Today, many patients with periodontal disease show tooth positioning that compromises their ability to properly mechanically sanitise all tooth surfaces. With appropriate interdisciplinary periodontal-orthodontic treatment, it is possible to re-establish a healthy and functional dentition. However, while orthodontic treatment can realign periodontally affected teeth, the aesthetic appearance can be compromised by gingival recession secondary to this, due to dehiscences or fenestrations of the alveolar bone in combination with a thin gingival phenotype[10, 17, 20].

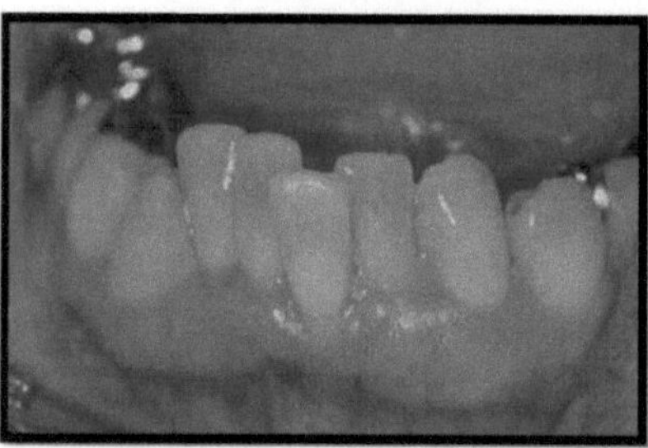
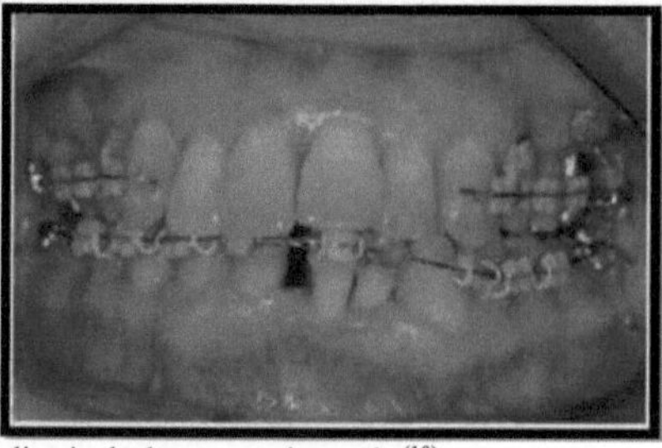

Figure XXVI: Initial clinical situation, with dental crowding in the lower anterior teeth. [10]
Figure XXVII: orthodontic treatment, including the placement of a micro-implant in the area of tooth #25.[10]

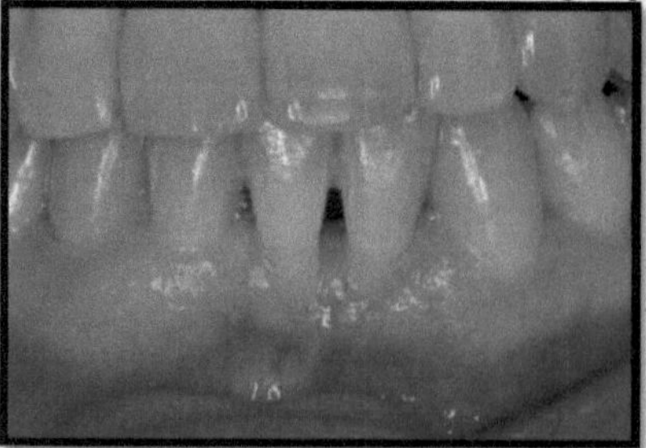

Figure XXVIII: clinical situation after orthodontic treatment, showing gingival recessions on teeth #32 and #41. [10]
Modern concepts in dentistry emphasise the etiological significance of biological, systemic and pro-

inflammatory mediators in the development of periodontal disease. Goldman et al. (1990) explained that malocclusion and the abnormal positioning of teeth are now recognised as potentially contributing factors to the course of the disease when they cause occlusal trauma: excessive functional stress can initiate inflammatory changes in the periodontium and thus enhance the destructive processes of bacteria[78].

Geiger (2001) analysed the scientific literature in order to assess whether or not malocclusion is an etiological factor in periodontal disease. A positive correlation was found between posterior teeth with abnormal axial mesiodistal inclinations, as well as those that experienced migration phenomena, and periodontal destruction. Orthodontic correction of mesially inclined molars with attachment loss should be part of periodontal therapy in order to promote their maintenance in the dental arches. In extreme cases of vertical overbite, direct trauma to the gums caused by the incisal edges of the mandibular incisors can result in palatal gingival recession of the maxillary incisors. In class II division 2 malocclusions with maxillary incisor linguoversion, functional trauma can cause marginal gingival recession of the labial gingiva of the mandibular incisors. When dental crowding leads to adjacent teeth overlapping, the interproximal space can be minimal and there can be greater proximity of the roots, which constitutes a bad environment for tissue health due to the difficulty in removing plaque and subgingival calculus in the interproximal spaces. In full-mouth occlusion of maxillary molars and lingual occlusion of their opponents, excessive occlusal stress can result in occlusal trauma; if there is inflammation, greater loss of adherence can occur[78].

Experiments carried out on both humans and animals have shown convincing evidence that neither unilateral forces nor alternating forces applied to a healthy periodontium result in the formation of periodontal pockets or loss of connective tissue insertion. Occlusal trauma cannot induce the destruction of periodontal tissues, but it can cause a resorption of alveolar bone, leading to an increase in tooth mobility, which can be transient or permanent. This bone resorption should be seen as a physiological adaptation of the periodontal ligament and alveolar bone to traumatic forces. In teeth with periodontal disease associated with plaque, occlusal trauma can, under certain conditions, act as a co-factor in the destructive process of the disease, increasing its speed of progression[5].

Mucogingival defects, especially of the mandibular incisors, and the development of localised gingival recession, have been related to the following aetiological factors, individually or in combination: minimal adhered gingiva; thin labial alveolar bone; severe labial inclination; alveolar bone fenestration; occlusal trauma. It therefore seems prudent to carry out an orthodontic intervention prior to periodontal surgical treatment, which improves the anatomical and functional environment, as it can limit gingival recession and, in some cases, induce creeping reattachment or spontaneous reattachment[10, 20, 74, 78].

CHAPTER 4

CONCLUSION

Gingival recessions are one of the main complaints of dental patients. There is a wide variety of mucogingival surgical techniques, which are quite predictable and produce satisfactory solutions for treating this problem. However, complete root coverage is not always achievable, even if gingival recession is not associated with loss of adhesion and interproximal bone. The selection of the appropriate procedure, a precise and meticulous surgical technique and a careful analysis of the patient's risk and prognostic factors will, from the outset, produce predictable and successful clinical results, making root coverage surgery an effective periodontal therapy for the treatment of gingival recessions.

Although most of the benchmarks for the prognosis and outcome of root coverage surgery are scientifically well-founded enough to qualify as such, there is a need for more scientific research to counteract some of the empiricism in the clinical practice of this procedure:

- Root straightening in teeth with prominent roots or very pronounced convexities has no parameters or reference values for root wear;
- There is insufficient information on the influence of systemic diseases on graft and soft tissue flap healing and, consequently, on the admission of patients to clinical trials of root coverage surgical techniques;
- It has not yet been possible to define values for the width of the gingival recession and the dimensions of the intraosseous defect at which the outcome of mucogingival surgery may be compromised;
- There is no reference value for the depth of the vestibule and the presence of muscle insertions close to the gingival margin for the prognosis of root coverage surgery.

CHAPTER 5

BIBLIOGRAPHY

1.   Lang NP, Adler R, Joss A, Nyman S. Absence of bleeding on probing. An indicator of periodontal stability. Journal of clinical periodontology. 1990;17(10):714-21. Epub 1990/11/01.

2.   Pini Prato GP, Baldi C, Nieri M, Franseschi D, Cortellini P, Clauser C, et al. Coronally advanced flap: the post-surgical position of the gingival margin is an important factor for achieving complete root coverage. Journal of periodontology. 2005;76(5):713-22. Epub 2005/05/19.

3.   Zucchelli G, Testori T, De Sanctis M. Clinical and anatomical factors limiting treatment outcomes of gingival recession: a new method to predetermine the line of root coverage. Journal of periodontology. 2006;77(4):714-21. Epub 2006/04/06.

4.   Muller HP, Eger T. Masticatory mucosa and periodontal phenotype: a review. The International journal of periodontics & restorative dentistry. 2002;22(2):172-83. Epub 2002/05/22.

5.   Lindhe JK, T.; Lang, N. P. Clinical periodontology and implant dentistry. 4th ed. Rio de Janeiro: Guanabara Koogan; 2005. 1013 p.

6.   Antonieta de Queiroz Côrtes AWS, Marcio Z. Casati, Francisco H. Nociti Jr., Enilson A. Sallum. A two-year prospective study of coronally positioned flap with or without acellular dermal matrix graft. Journal of clinical periodontology. 2006;33:683-9.

7.   Angela Guimarães Martins DCA, Antonio Wilson Sallum, Enilson A. Sallum, Márcio Z. Casati, Francisco H. Smoking May Affect Root Coverage Outcome: A Prospective Clinical Study in Humans. Journal of periodontology. 2004;75:586-91.

8.   Cortellini P, Pini Prato G. Coronally advanced flap and combination therapy for root coverage. Clinical strategies based on scientific evidence and clinical experience. Periodontology 2000. 2012;59(1):158-84. Epub 2012/04/18.

9.   Deliberador TM, Bosco AF, Martins TM, Nagata MJ. Treatment of gingival recessions associated with cervical abrasion lesions with subepithelial connective tissue graft: a case report. European journal of dentistry. 2009;3(4):318-23. Epub 2009/10/15.

10.   Kasaj A, Wehrbein H, Gortan-Kasaj A, Reichert C, Willershausen B. Interdisciplinary approach for the treatment of periodontally compromised malpositioned anterior teeth: a case report.

Cases journal. 2009;2:8568. Epub 2009/10/16.

11.   Miller PD, Jr. A classification of marginal tissue recession. The International journal of periodontics & restorative dentistry. 1985;5(2):8-13. Epub 1985/01/01.

12.   Bouchard P, Malet J, Borghetti A. Decision-making in aesthetics: root coverage revisited. Periodontology 2000. 2001;27:97-120. Epub 2001/09/12.

13.   Holbrook T, Ochsenbein C. Complete coverage of the denuded root surface with a one-stage gingival graft. The International journal of periodontics & restorative dentistry. 1983;3(3):8-27. Epub 1983/01/01.

14.   de Sanctis M, Zucchelli G. Coronally advanced flap: a modified surgical approach for isolated recession-type defects: three-year results. Journal of clinical periodontology. 2007;34(3):262-8. Epub 2007/02/21.

15.   Otero-Cagide FJ, Otero-Cagide MF. Unique creeping attachment after autogenous gingival grafting: case report. J Can Dent Assoc. 2003;69(7):432-5. Epub 2003/07/26.

16.   Zucchelli G, Mele M, Stefanini M, Mazzotti C, Mounssif I, Marzadori M, et al. Predetermination of root coverage. Journal of periodontology. 2010;81(7):1019-26. Epub 2010/03/03.

17.   Gray JL. When Not to Perform Root Coverage Procedures. Journal of periodontology. 2000;71(6):1048-9.

18.   Goldstein M, Brayer L, Schwartz Z. A critical evaluation of methods for root coverage. Critical reviews in oral biology and medicine : an official publication of the American Association of Oral Biologists. 1996;7(1):87-98. Epub 1996/01/01.

19.   Leake JM, J. Treatment of Gingival Recession: An Analysis of Current Literature and Recommendations. Community 300Y.

20.   Saygun I KS, Ozdemir A, Sagdiç D. Multidisciplinary Treatment Approach for the Localised Gingival Recession: A Case Report. Turk J Med Sci. 2005;35:57-63.

21.   Pagliaro U, Nieri M, Franceschi D, Clauser C, Pini-Prato G. Evidence-based mucogingival therapy. Part 1: A critical review of the literature on root coverage procedures. Journal of periodontology. 2003;74(5):709-40. Epub 2003/06/21.

22.   Wennstrom JL. Mucogingival considerations in orthodontic treatment. Seminars in orthodontics. 1996;2(1):46-54. Epub 1996/03/01.

23.   Zucchelli G, De Sanctis M. Treatment of multiple recession-type defects in patients with esthetic demands. Journal of periodontology. 2000;71(9):1506-14. Epub 2000/10/07.

24.   Chambrone L, Lima LA, Pustiglioni FE, Chambrone LA. Systematic review of periodontal plastic surgery in the treatment of multiple recession-type defects. J Can Dent Assoc. 2009;75(3):203a-f. Epub 2009/04/10.

25.   Chambrone L, Chambrone LA. Gingival recessions caused by lip piercing: case report. Dent Assist. 2004;73(5):14, 6-7, 9. Epub 2004/11/24.

26.   Peres MF, Ribeiro Edel P, Bittencourt S, Sallum EA, Sallum AW, Nociti-Junior FH, et al. Influence of crown shape on root coverage therapy. Journal of applied oral science : FOB magazine. 2009;17(4):330-4. Epub 2009/08/12.

27.   Padbury A JE, R; Wang, HL. Interactions between the gingiva and the margin of restorations. Journal of clinical periodontology. 2003;30:379-85.

28.   Vandana KV, KV. Periodontal regeneration in vital and nonvital teeh - A clinical study. Endodontology. 2003;15:26-32.

29.   Wennstrom JL, Zucchelli G. Increased gingival dimensions. A significant factor for successful outcome of root coverage procedures? A 2-year prospective clinical study. Journal of clinical periodontology. 1996;23(8):770-7. Epub 1996/08/01.

30.   Prato GP, Rotundo R, Magnani C, Ficarra G. Viral etiology of gingival recession. A case report. Journal of periodontology. 2002;73(1):110-4. Epub 2002/02/16.

31.   Bruno JF. Connective tissue graft technique assuring wide root coverage. The International journal of periodontics & restorative dentistry. 1994;14(2):126-37. Epub 1994/04/01.

32.   Silva CO, Sallum AW, de Lima AF, Tatakis DN. Coronally positioned flap for root coverage: poorer outcomes in smokers. Journal of periodontology. 2006;77(1):81-7. Epub 2006/04/04.

33.   Tenenbaum H. A clinical study comparing the width of attached gingiva and the prevalence of gingival recessions. Journal of clinical periodontology. 1982;9(1):86-92. Epub 1982/01/01.

34.   M. Del Pizzo GZ, F. Modica, R. Villa, C. Debernardi. Coronally advanced flap with or without enamel matrix derivative for root coverage: a 2-year study. Journal of clinical periodontology. 2005;32:1181-7.

35.   Nieri M, Rotundo R, Franceschi D, Cairo F, Cortellini P, Pini Prato G. Factors affecting the outcome of the coronally advanced flap procedure: a Bayesian network analysis. Journal of

periodontology. 2009;80(3):405-10. Epub 2009/03/04.

36.		Pini Prato G, Rotundo R, Franceschi D, Cairo F, Cortellini P, Nieri M. Fourteen-year outcomes of coronally advanced flap for root coverage: follow-up from a randomised trial. Journal of clinical periodontology. 2011;38(8):715-20. Epub 2011/06/04.

37.		Paolantonio M, Dolci M, Esposito P, D'Archivio D, Lisanti L, Di Luccio A, et al. Subpedicle acellular dermal matrix graft and autogenous connective tissue graft in the treatment of gingival recessions: a comparative 1-year clinical study. Journal of periodontology. 2002;73(11):1299-307. Epub 2002/12/14.

38.		Woodyard JG, Greenwell H, Hill M, Drisko C, Iasella JM, Scheetz J. The clinical effect of acellular dermal matrix on gingival thickness and root coverage compared to coronally positioned flap alone. Journal of periodontology. 2004;75(1):44-56. Epub 2004/03/18.

39.		Moriyama T, Matsumoto S, Makiishi T. Root coverage technique with enamel matrix derivative. The Bulletin of Tokyo Dental College. 2009;50(2):97-104. Epub 2009/10/10.

40.		Chambrone L, Sukekava F, Araujo MG, Pustiglioni FE, Chambrone LA, Lima LA. Root-coverage procedures for the treatment of localised recession-type defects: a Cochrane systematic review. Journal of periodontology. 2010;81(4):452-78. Epub 2010/04/07.

41.		Camargo PMM, P. R.; Kenney, E. B. The use of free gingival grafts for aesthetic purposes. Periodontology 2000. 2001;27:72-96.

42.		Wang HL, Bunyaratavej P, Labadie M, Shyr Y, MacNeil RL. Comparison of 2 clinical techniques for treatment of gingival recession. Journal of periodontology. 2001;72(10):1301- 11. Epub 2001/11/09.

43.		Rosetti EP, Marcantonio RA, Rossa C, Jr, Chaves ES, Goissis G, Marcantonio E, Jr. Treatment of gingival recession: comparative study between subepithelial connective tissue graft and guided tissue regeneration. Journal of periodontology. 2000;71(9):1441-7. Epub 2000/10/07.

44.		Abolfazli N, Saleh-Saber F, Eskandari A, Lafzi A. A comparative study of the long term results of root coverage with connective tissue graft or enamel matrix protein: 24- month results. Medicina oral, patologia oral y cirugia bucal. 2009;14(6):E304-9. Epub 2009/03/21.

45.		Nickles K, Ratka-Kruger P, Neukranz E, Raetzke P, Eickholz P. Ten-year results after connective tissue grafts and guided tissue regeneration for root coverage. Journal of periodontology. 2010;81(6):827-36. Epub 2010/05/11.

46.   John R. Dodge HG, Connie Drisko, John W. Wittwer, John Yancey, George Rebitski. Improved Bone Regeneration and Root Coverage Using a Resorbable Membrane with Physically Assisted Cell Migration and DFDBA. The International journal of periodontics & restorative dentistry. 2000;20:398-411.

47.   Paolantonio M. Treatment of gingival recessions by combined periodontal regenerative technique, guided tissue regeneration, and subpedicle connective tissue graft. A comparative clinical study. Journal of periodontology. 2002;73(1):53-62. Epub 2002/02/16.

48.   Miller PD, Jr. Regenerative and reconstructive periodontal plastic surgery. Mucogingival surgery. Dental clinics of North America. 1988;32(2):287-306. Epub 1988/04/01.

49.   Joly JC, Carvalho AM, da Silva RC, Ciotti DL, Cury PR. Root coverage in isolated gingival recessions using autograft versus allograft: a pilot study. Journal of periodontology. 2007;78(6):1017-22. Epub 2007/06/02.

50.   Saletta DPP, G; Pagliaro, U; Baldi, C; Mauri, M; Nieri, M. Coronally Advanced Flap Procedure: Is the Interdental Papilla a Prognostic Factor for Root Coverage? Journal of periodontology. 2001;72(6):760-6.

51.   Cortellini P, Carnevale G, Sanz M, Tonetti MS. Treatment of deep and shallow intrabony defects. A multicentre randomized controlled clinical trial. Journal of clinical periodontology. 1998;25(12):981-7. Epub 1998/12/30.

52.   Cortellini P, Tonetti MS. Evaluation of the effect of tooth vitality on regenerative outcomes in infrabony defects. Journal of clinical periodontology. 2001;28(7):672-9. Epub 2001/06/26.

53.   Zucchelli G, Mele M, Stefanini M, Mazzotti C, Marzadori M, Montebugnoli L, et al. Patient morbidity and root coverage outcome after subepithelial connective tissue and de- epithelialised grafts: a comparative randomized-controlled clinical trial. Journal of clinical periodontology. 2010;37(8):728-38. Epub 2010/07/02.

54.   Henriques PS, Pelegrine AA, Nogueira AA, Borghi MM. Application of subepithelial connective tissue graft with or without enamel matrix derivative for root coverage: a split-mouth randomised study. Journal of oral science. 2010;52(3):463-71. Epub 2010/10/01.

55.   Berlucchi I, Francetti L, Del Fabbro M, Basso M, Weinstein RL. The influence of anatomical features on the outcome of gingival recessions treated with coronally advanced flap and enamel matrix derivative: a 1-year prospective study. Journal of periodontology. 2005;76(6):899-907. Epub 2005/06/14.

56.   Thomas S. Barker MAC, Francisco Rivera-Hidalgo, M. Miles Beach, Jeffrey A. Rossmann, David G. Kerns, T. Bradley Crump, Jay D. Shulman. A Comparative Study of Root Coverage Using Two Different Acellular Dermal Matrix Products. Journal of periodontology. 2010;81:1596-603.

57.   Hansmeier U, Eickholz P. Effect of root coverage on oral health impact profile (g49): a pilot study. International journal of dentistry. 2010;2010:252303. Epub 2010/07/16.

58.   Esteibar JR, Zorzano LA, Cundin EE, Blanco JD, Medina JR. Complete root coverage of Miller Class III recessions. The International journal of periodontics & restorative dentistry. 2011;31(4):e1-7. Epub 2011/08/13.

59.   Zucchelli G, De Sanctis M. The coronally advanced flap for the treatment of multiple recession defects: a modified surgical approach for the upper anterior teeth. Journal of the International Academy of Periodontology. 2007;9(3):96-103. Epub 2007/08/25.

60.   Pini Prato G, Pagliaro U, Baldi C, Nieri M, Saletta D, Cairo F, et al. Coronally advanced flap procedure for root coverage. Flap with tension versus flap without tension: a randomised controlled clinical study. Journal of periodontology. 2000;71(2):188-201. Epub 2000/03/11.

61.   Baldi C, Pini-Prato G, Pagliaro U, Nieri M, Saletta D, Muzzi L, et al. Coronally advanced flap procedure for root coverage. Is flap thickness a relevant predictor to achieve root coverage? A 19-case series. Journal of periodontology. 1999;70(9):1077-84. Epub 1999/10/03.

62.   Cheng YF, Chen JW, Lin SJ, Lu HK. Is coronally positioned flap procedure adjunct with enamel matrix derivative or root conditioning a relevant predictor for achieving root coverage? A systemic review. Journal of periodontal research. 2007;42(5):474-85. Epub 2007/09/01.

63.   Cairo F, Nieri M, Cattabriga M, Cortellini P, De Paoli S, De Sanctis M, et al. Root coverage aesthetic score after treatment of gingival recession: an interrater agreement multicentre study. Journal of periodontology. 2010;81(12):1752-8. Epub 2010/07/16.

64.   Chambrone L, Sukekava F, Araujo MG, Pustiglioni FE, Chambrone LA, Lima LA. Root coverage procedures for the treatment of localised recession-type defects. Cochrane Database Syst Rev. 2009(2):CD007161. Epub 2009/04/17.

65.   Kassab MM, Badawi H, Dentino AR. Treatment of gingival recession. Dental clinics of North America. 2010;54(1):129-40. Epub 2010/01/28.

66.   Quinones CR. Treatment of gingival recession using guided periodontal tissue regeneration. Practical periodontics and aesthetic dentistry : PPAD. 1997;9(2):145-53; quiz 54. Epub 1997/03/01.

67.   Blanc A, Pare-Dargent C, Giovannoli JL. [Treatment of gingival recession with a coronally

repositioned flap.] Journal de parodontologie. 1991;10(3):329-34. Epub 1991/09/01. Traitement des recessions gingivales par lambeau positionne coronairement.

68.   Tozum TF, Keceli HG, Guncu GN, Hatipoglu H, Sengun D. Treatment of gingival recession: comparison of two techniques of subepithelial connective tissue graft. Journal of periodontology. 2005;76(11):1842-8. Epub 2005/11/09.

69.   Kerner S, Borghetti A, Katsahian S, Etienne D, Malet J, Mora F, et al. A retrospective study of root coverage procedures using an image analysis system. Journal of clinical periodontology. 2008;35(4):346-55. Epub 2008/03/21.

70.   Clauser C, Nieri M, Franceschi D, Pagliaro U, Pini-Prato G. Evidence-based mucogingival therapy. Part 2: Ordinary and individual patient data meta-analyses of surgical treatment of recession using complete root coverage as the outcome variable. Journal of periodontology. 2003;74(5):741-56. Epub 2003/06/21.

71.   Klein F, Kim TS, Hassfeld S, Staehle HJ, Reitmeir P, Holle R, et al. Radiographic defect depth and width for prognosis and description of periodontal healing of infrabony defects. Journal of periodontology. 2001;72(12):1639-46. Epub 2002/01/29.

72.   Kassab MM, Cohen RE. Treatment of gingival recession. J Am Dent Assoc. 2002;133(11):1499-506; quiz 540. Epub 2002/12/05.

73.   Hwang D, Wang HL. Flap thickness as a predictor of root coverage: a systematic review. Journal of periodontology. 2006;77(10):1625-34. Epub 2006/10/13.

74.   Deepa D, Mehta DS, Puri VK, Shetty S. Combined periodontic- orthodonticendodontic interdisciplinary approach in the treatment of periodontally compromised tooth. Journal of Indian Society of Periodontology. 2010;14(2):139-43. Epub 2010/04/01.

75.   Flores-Mir C. Does orthodontic treatment lead to gingival recession? Evidence- based dentistry. 2011;12(1):20. Epub 2011/03/26.

76.   Melsen B. Tissue reaction to orthodontic tooth movement--a new paradigm. European journal of orthodontics. 2001;23(6):671-81. Epub 2002/03/14.

77.   Santamaria MP, Ambrosano GM, Casati MZ, Nociti FH, Jr., Sallum AW, Sallum EA. The influence of local anatomy on the outcome of treatment of gingival recession associated with non-carious cervical lesions. Journal of periodontology. 2010;81(7):1027-34. Epub 2010/03/11.

78.   Geiger AM. Malocclusion as an etiologic factor in periodontal disease: a retrospective essay.

American journal of orthodontics and dentofacial orthopedics : official publication of the American Association of Orthodontists, its constituent societies, and the American Board of Orthodontics. 2001;120(2):112-5.